Survivors

Survívors

Experiences of Childhood
Sexual Abuse and Healing

by Khristine Hopkins

Celestial Arts
Berkeley, California

Celestial Arts
P.O. Box 7123
Berkeley, California 94707

Cover design by Fifth Street Design

Text design by Victor Ichioka

Library of Congress Cataloging-in-Publication Data

Hopkins, Khristine.
    Survivors : experiences of childhood sexual abuse & Healing /
  by Khristine Hopkins
        p.   cm.
     ISBN 0-89087-711-4 : $14.95
     1. Adult child sexual abuse victims—Portraits. 2. Adult child
  sexual abuse victims.   I. Title
RC569.5.A28H67   1994
616.85'8369—dc20   94-5961
                                CIP

First Printing, 1994

1 2 3 4 5 / 98 97 96 95 94

For Donald and Maximillian Beal

To flee from memory

had we the wings,

many would fly.

—Emily Dickinson

Contents

Preface

I am a photographer. My artwork has always reflected my personal life. I am also a survivor of childhood sexual abuse.

The connection between art and life became a crucial one eight years ago when painful memories began to surface around the time that my son was born. Not remembering until later in life is a common experience for survivors of traumatic events. When I joined a short-term therapy group for women survivors of childhood sexual abuse, I became completely blocked as an artist.

My husband, a painter, believed that I could overcome the block if I processed my experience through my artwork. So I made a decision to use visual metaphors and words to work through the feelings that were emerging.

My first photograph was of my son Max who was three at the time. I wanted to capture something about the vulnerability of children and the fragility of their boundaries. A careless person can cross those boundaries and cause untold suffering. As I put together the exhibit, this photograph took on more levels of meaning for me. As the first piece in the show, its purpose has been to help viewers make the connection between adults in the photographs and the children they once were.

The next photograph, a self-portrait, was about my relationship with my father. Making these initial photographs comforted me at a time when I was in much pain and led me to ask the other women in the group to collaborate. We felt it was important that each of us appear in at least one photograph about the abuse experience and another about the healing process. The visual metaphors express what is particular to our own experience, but they also function as archetypes. So a pregnant, unnamed survivor in the last photograph of the exhibit, stands for triumph over shame. As things began to take shape, we started to work together on the text for the photographs and the scope and goals of the project became more defined. The hand-coloring and the small size of the photographs help to draw the viewer into the intimate circle of these women.

Although childhood sexual abuse affects people of every race, and class, and gender, this exhibit does not attempt to reflect that diversity. It represents the experience of a small group of women, but, hopefully, it will touch many others.

The photographs are not graphic depictions of abuse. I'm interested in enlightening and healing rather than in shocking people. I knew that these photographs would bring up pain, for those of us in the project, and for many viewers. However, after evoking this pain, I didn't want to leave people feeling hopeless. The photographs do not only express pain, but also the incredible strength of these women ... and through this strength lies hope. The belief that healing is possible transforms a victim into a survivor.

Acknowledgments

I would like to thank the many people who have helped with their time, efforts, and support since 1989 when I first conceived of this project. Unlike any exhibition I have had before, this one would never have been completed had it not been for enormous amounts of emotional support from my family, friends, and oftentimes complete strangers.

To Liddy, Nancy, Kaolin, Patsy, Yvonne, Mary, and Margit: No one has any idea of the courage that it takes to testify to such pain until they have done it. Hundreds of pages of comments left at each exhibition site bear witness to their committment to healing themselves, and the power of that committment to change the lives of others.

To the Artists Foundation of Boston's Volunteer Lawyers for the Arts Program for putting me in touch with Laurie Morin; her intelligence, perseverance, and warmth have made her an outstanding lawyer, agent, and friend.

To Dona Wheeler, my guide, and Alexandra Symonds for believing that the truth will set us free.

For childcare and friendship: Kaolin Davis, Diana Hardy, Leslie Eugenia, Lisa Rope, Candi McDonald, Amy Freeland, Jason Mauro, Linda Maloney, Nancy Schwarz, Gail Rapoza, Marian Roth, and Mary DeAngelis.

For help with the publishing maze: my editors Dave Hinds and Veronica Randall of Celestial Arts, Rev. Peter and Mrs. Ruth Fleck, Rachel Brown (Giese), Lucy Lovrien, Celia Chetham, Ruth Rogin, Gilbert Rogin, Ellen Bass, Laura Davis, Jackie Kelly, Karen Harding, Rob Read, Chris Seid, Charlotte Raymond, John Kerr, and my sister Lisa Orlando.

To Roslyn and David Goldway for their generosity in allowing me to build a darkroom in their home; to Joan and Al Marsh, Peggy and Boone Schirmer, and Kimble Stephens for allowing me to photograph in their homes.

For help with the exhibitions: (Wellfleet, Massachusetts) River Karmen, Ellen LeBow and Marla Freedman, owners of Hopkins Gallery, who gave these photographs their first chance to be seen and provided a safe environment for all of us, Bob Costa for his sensitivity toward the many people who found it difficult visiting this first showing, and Gayle Lovett for help hanging the show; (Provincetown, Massachusetts) Mary Spencer Nay of the Outermost Gallery, and Nancy Schwarz for help hanging the show; the Board of Directors of the Unitarian-Universalist Meeting House of Provincetown, and Rev. John Papandrew; (Windsor, Connecticut) Walter and Marilyn Rabetz of the Loomis Chaffe School; (Boston, Massachusetts) Ellen Graf of the Boston Public Library, Incest Resources at the Women's Center, Cambridge, Massachusetts, for providing literature and support for the BPL show, Anthony Fisher for help hanging the exhibit, Carolyn Rosenthal for housing, and Bruce Blaisdell for moral support; (Smith College, Northampton, Massachusetts) Charles Chetham of Provincetown, Chester Michalik, Katy Schneider and David Gloman of Northampton, Massachusetts; Bette Warner and Myrna Wierenga of the Cape Museum of Fine Arts, Dennis, Massachusetts; and Nick Capasso and Rachel Rosenfield Lafo of the DeCordova Museum, Lincoln, Massachusetts.

For material support: my husband, Donald Beal; LEF Foundation, Boston, Massachusetts and St. Helena, California; Orleans, Barnstable, and Provincetown Arts Lottery Councils and the Massachusetts Cultural Council; Puffin Foundation, Teaneck, New Jersey; and Lower Cape Citizens for Peaceful Alternatives.

For help with grant seeking: Betty Burkes, Arlene Toscano, and the Board of Directors of Independence House, Hyannis, Massachusetts; Elaine McIlroy and the staff of the Wellfleet Public Library; the staff of the Provincetown Public Library; Ruth Hill of the Schlesinger Library at Radcliffe College; Chris and Sarah Lutz; Judy Schaeffer, Catherine Bertulli, Bill Evaul, Marian Roth, Barbara Perry, Joan and Bob Holt, Sandy Longley, Danna Acker, Dr. Judith Alpert, Dr. Joan Smith, Ariane Tetrault, and Steve Terrini.

To Sandy Crosby for her clerical help and moral support; Mary Rehak and Ewa Nogiec-Smith for design and typesetting of announcements, signs, and text panels; and for technical help Marianne Maloney, Pat Bruno, Morgan Hayden and Mimi Thomas, Alyssa Hosford, and Rob DuToit.

Finally, there is no way to express the gratitude I feel toward my husband, Donald Beal for his belief in me even when I was ready to throw in the towel; and to my son Maximillian Beal for inspiring me to make these photographs and for sharing his childhood with me.

Prologue

OBSERVING, LOVING, AND

honoring the boundaries

of this particular child

provided the impetus for the

photographs which follow.

The children these adults

once were felt in need

of someone to speak for their

pain and grief. Now

they speak for themselves.

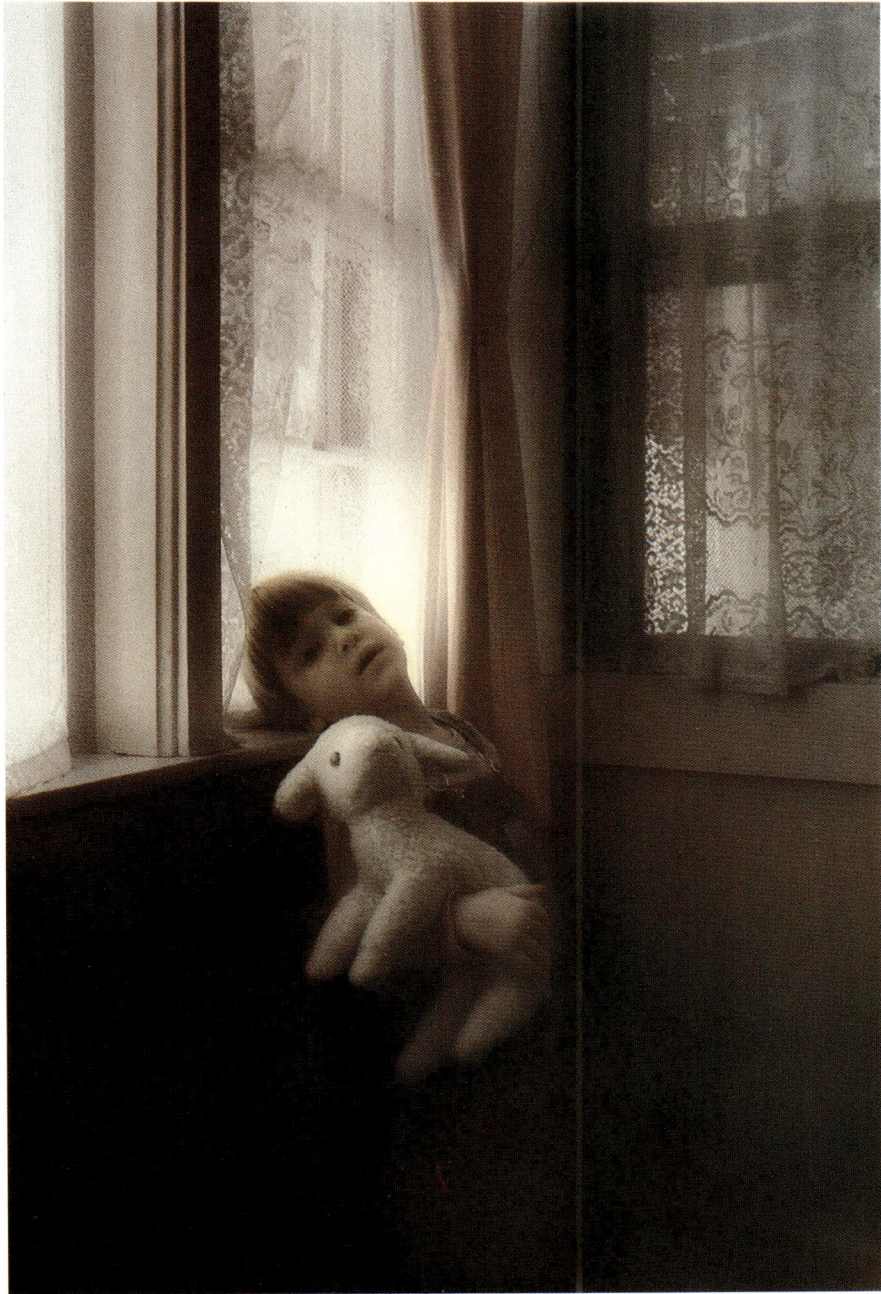

The Survivors

MARY

He's looking for me.

I close my eyes, block my ears,

and even hold my breath.

It's too late. He's found me.

I feel myself crying inside,

then and now.

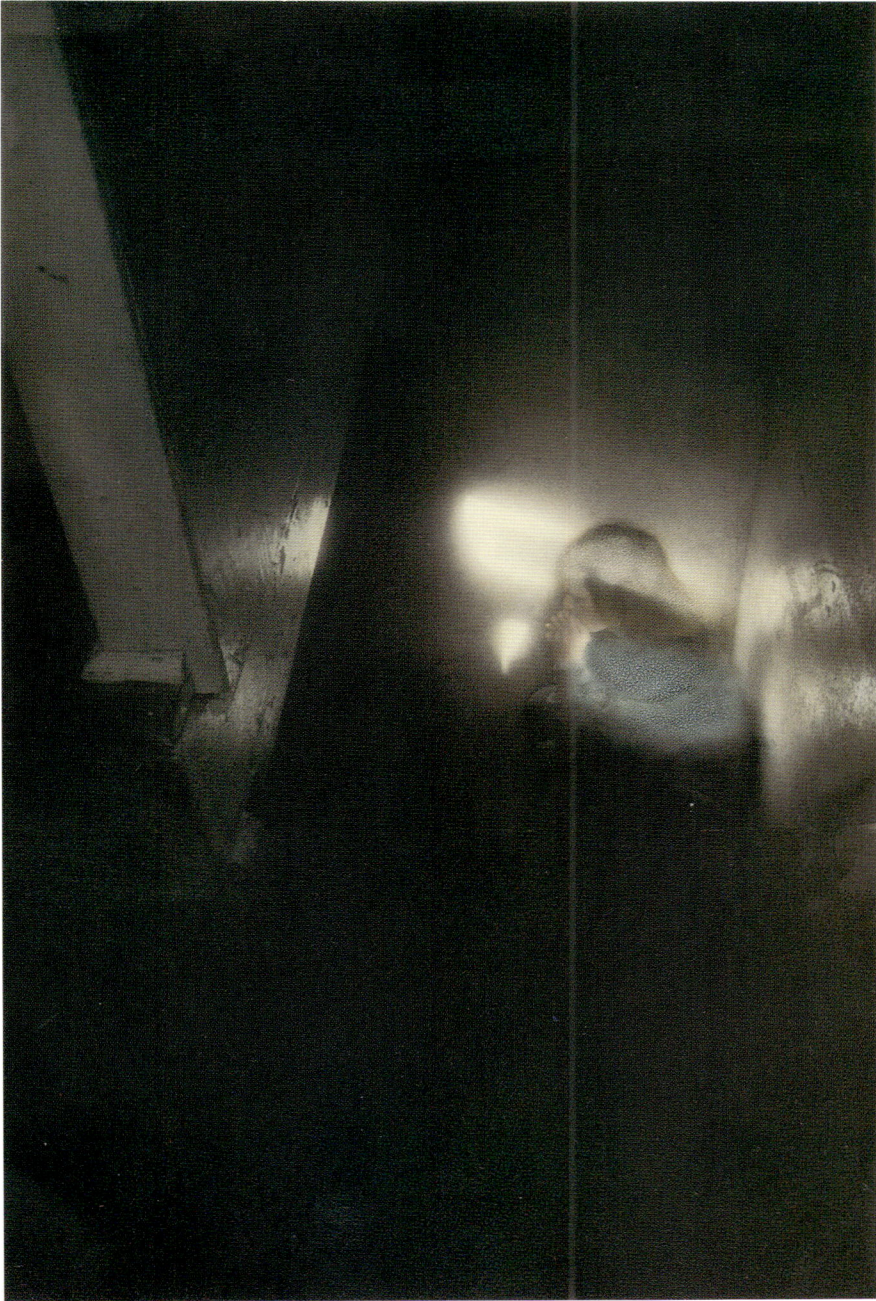

NANCY

HOW DID I FEEL?...

in pieces, fragmented, fearful

that I would never be able to

fit those pieces together—

this part wife, that part child,

never entirely myself,

never really whole.

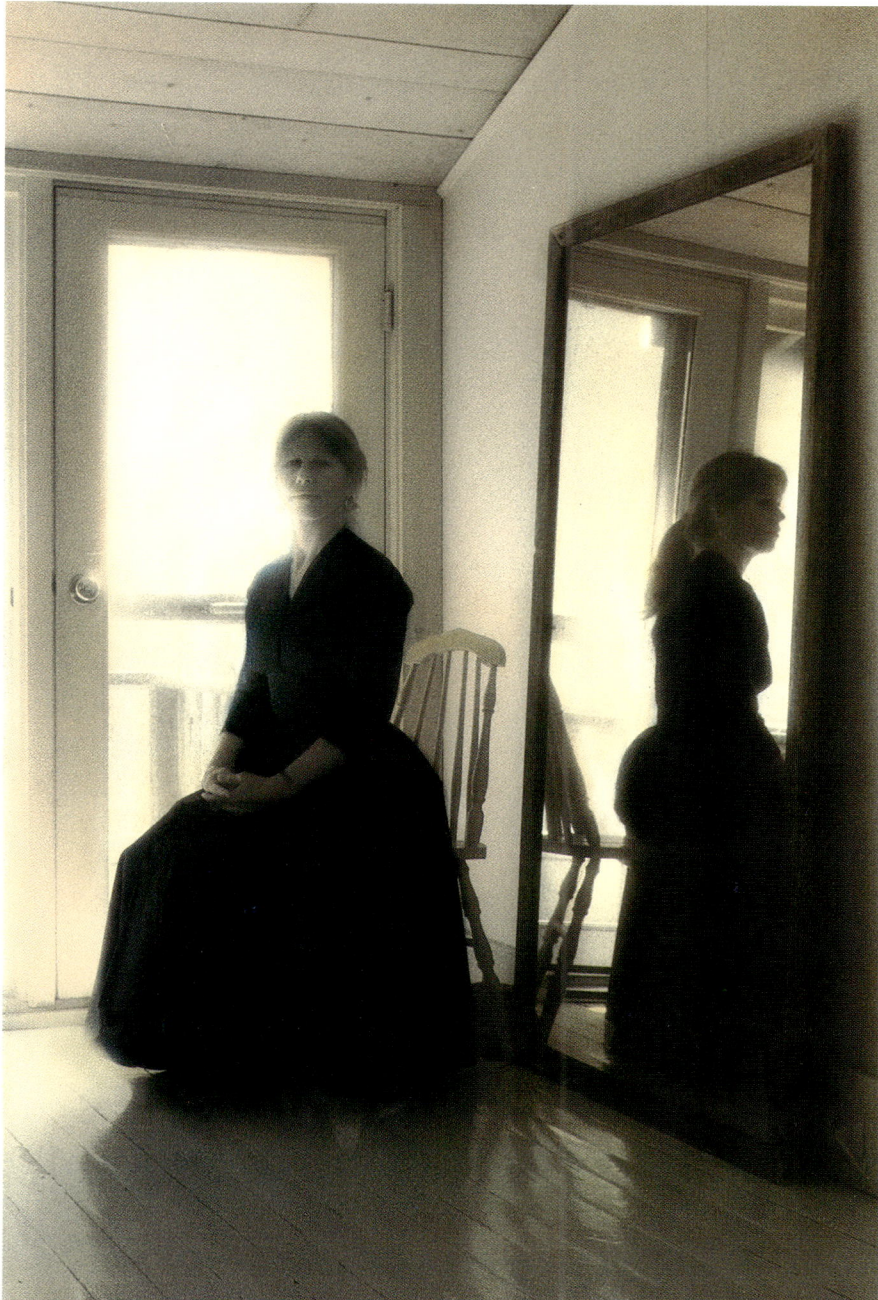

Liddy

I LEFT HOME AT EIGHTEEN

but I brought his voice with me.

It followed me relentlessly,

intruding and shaming me

in what should have been my

most private moments.

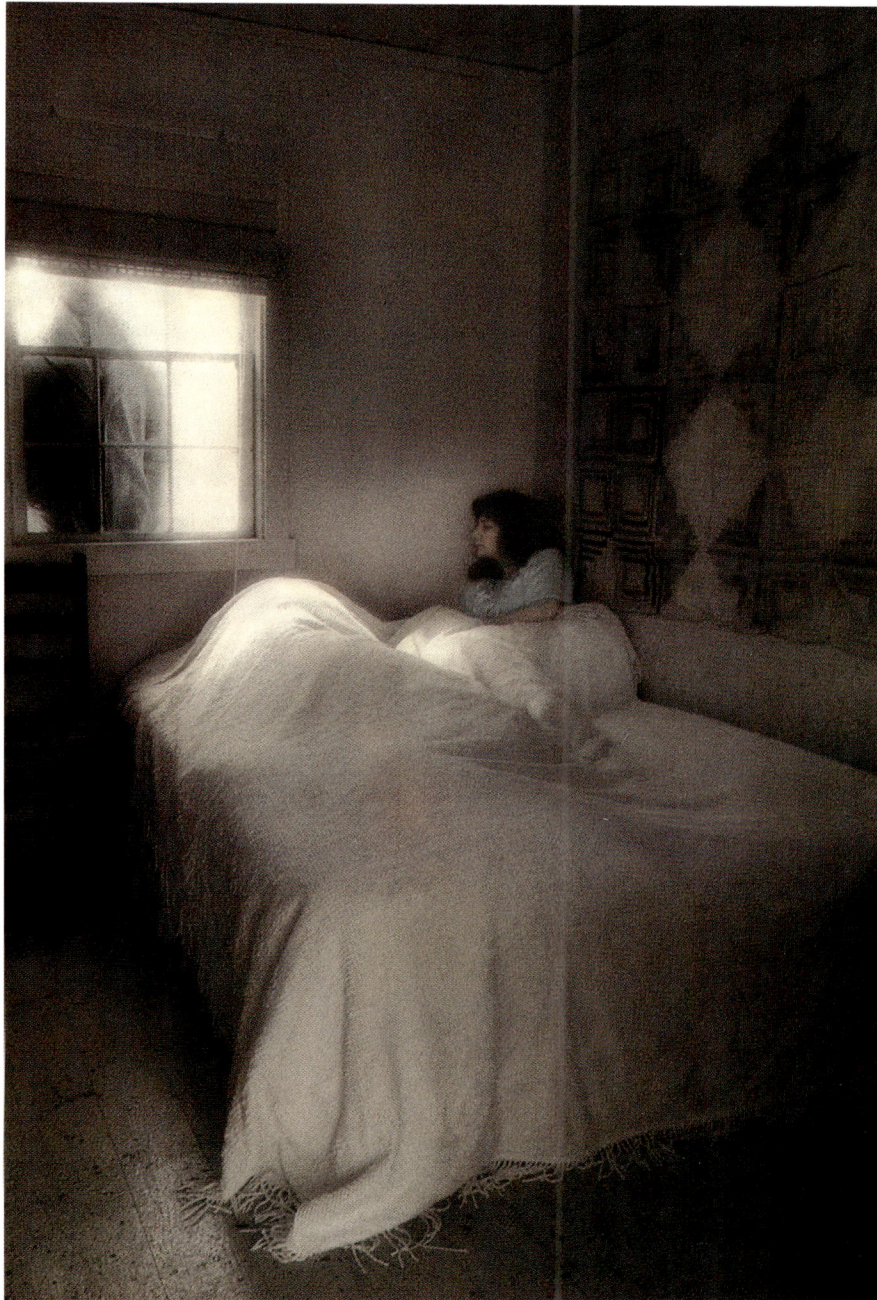

Khristine

It was hardly necessary

to drug me into submission.

Each childhood victimization

reinforced what I had learned

from my role in the family.

Those in power would prove

untrustworthy while I,

mute vessel, sat panic stricken,

quiescent.

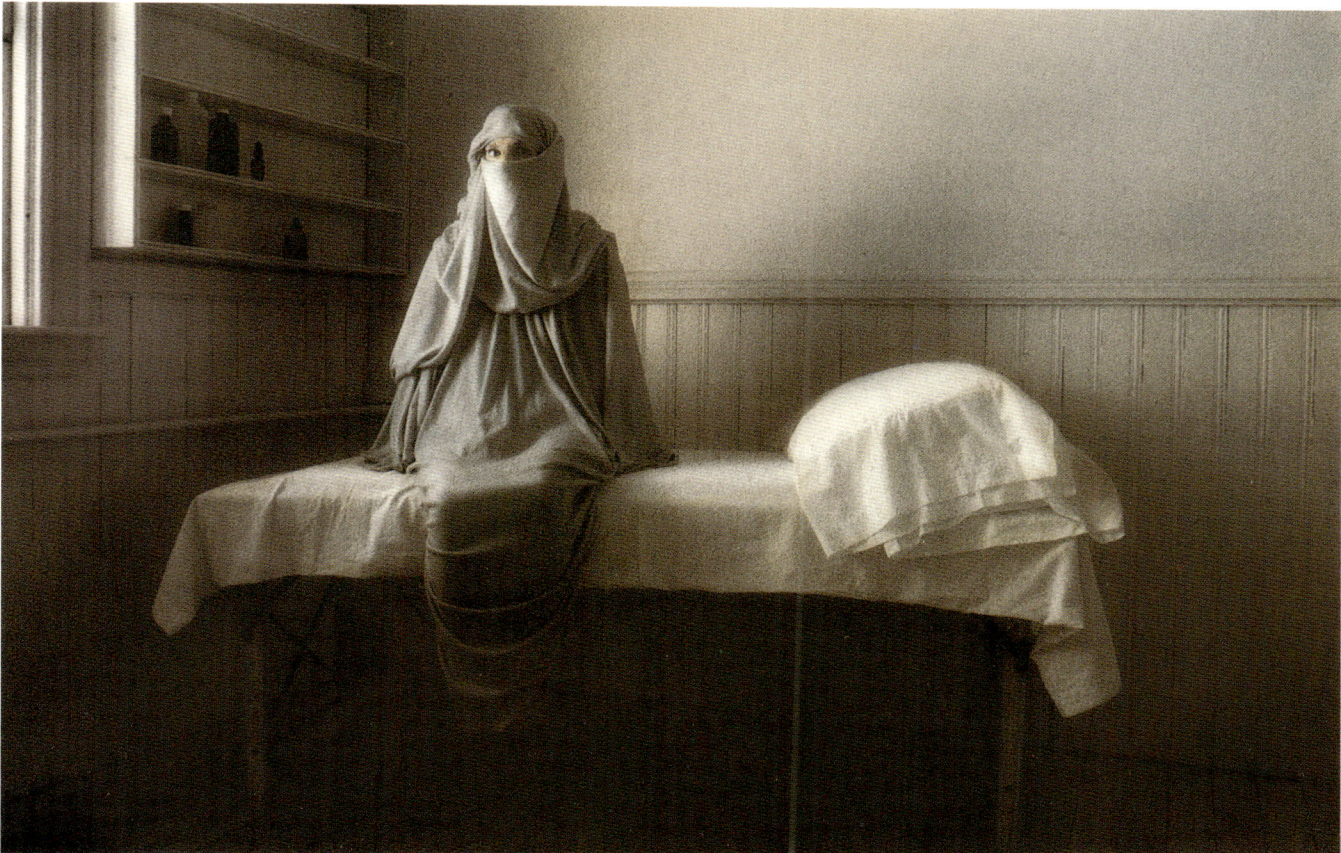

Nancy

As a result of my finally

remembering and speaking out

about my experience, I was

abandoned, isolated, and ostracized

by those from whom I had reason

to expect the most support.

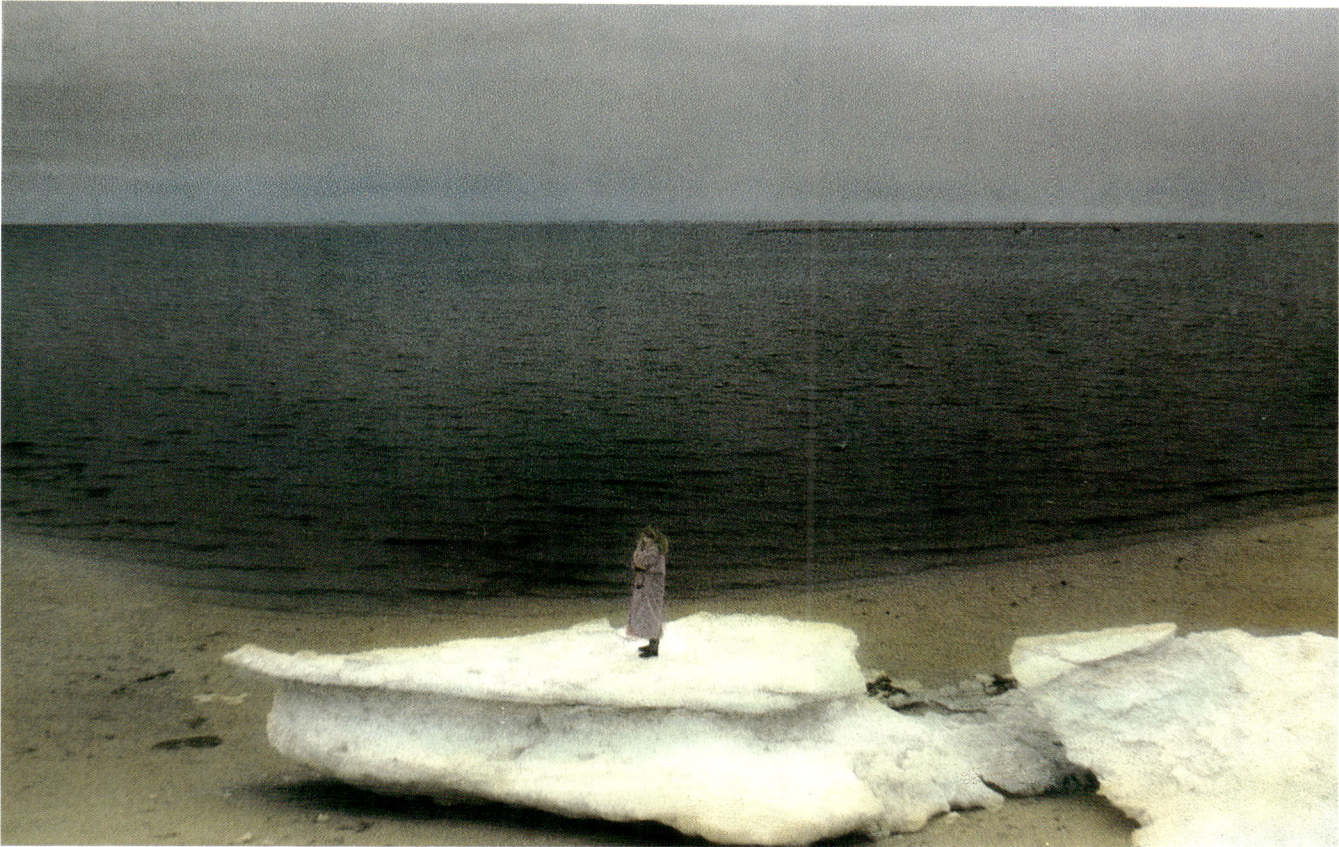

Patricia

I WAS RAPED WHEN I WAS

five years old by a group of

neighborhood boys.

Somewhere inside of me I think

I understood that what was to

follow would be even worse

than what had happened.

I was now perceived as

"damaged goods."

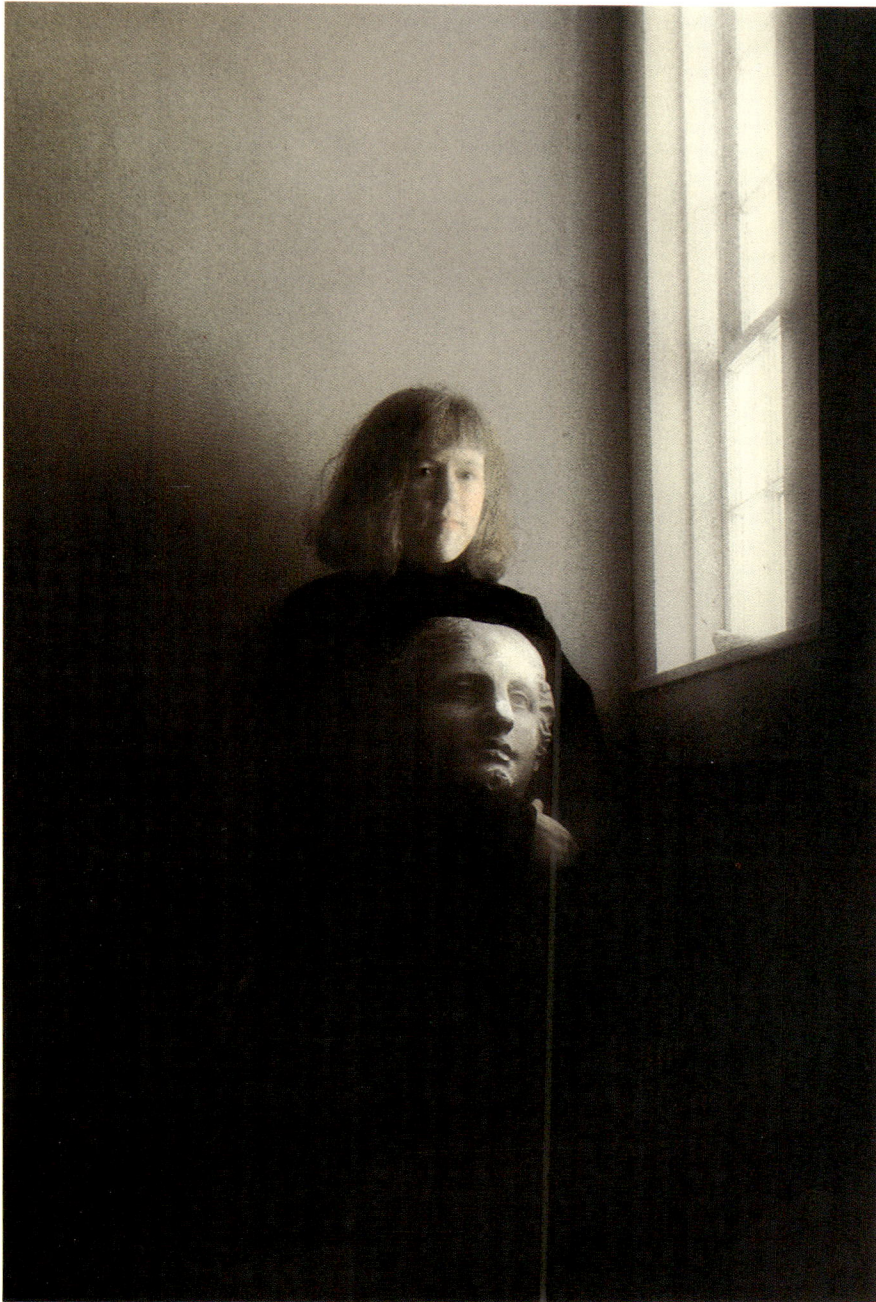

Yvonne

I AM DISEMBODIED...

split in two...the lower half

of me a woman's body,

frozen, waiting for deliverance...

the top half smaller, childlike,

full of despair...alienated

from my body, contaminated

in my spirit.

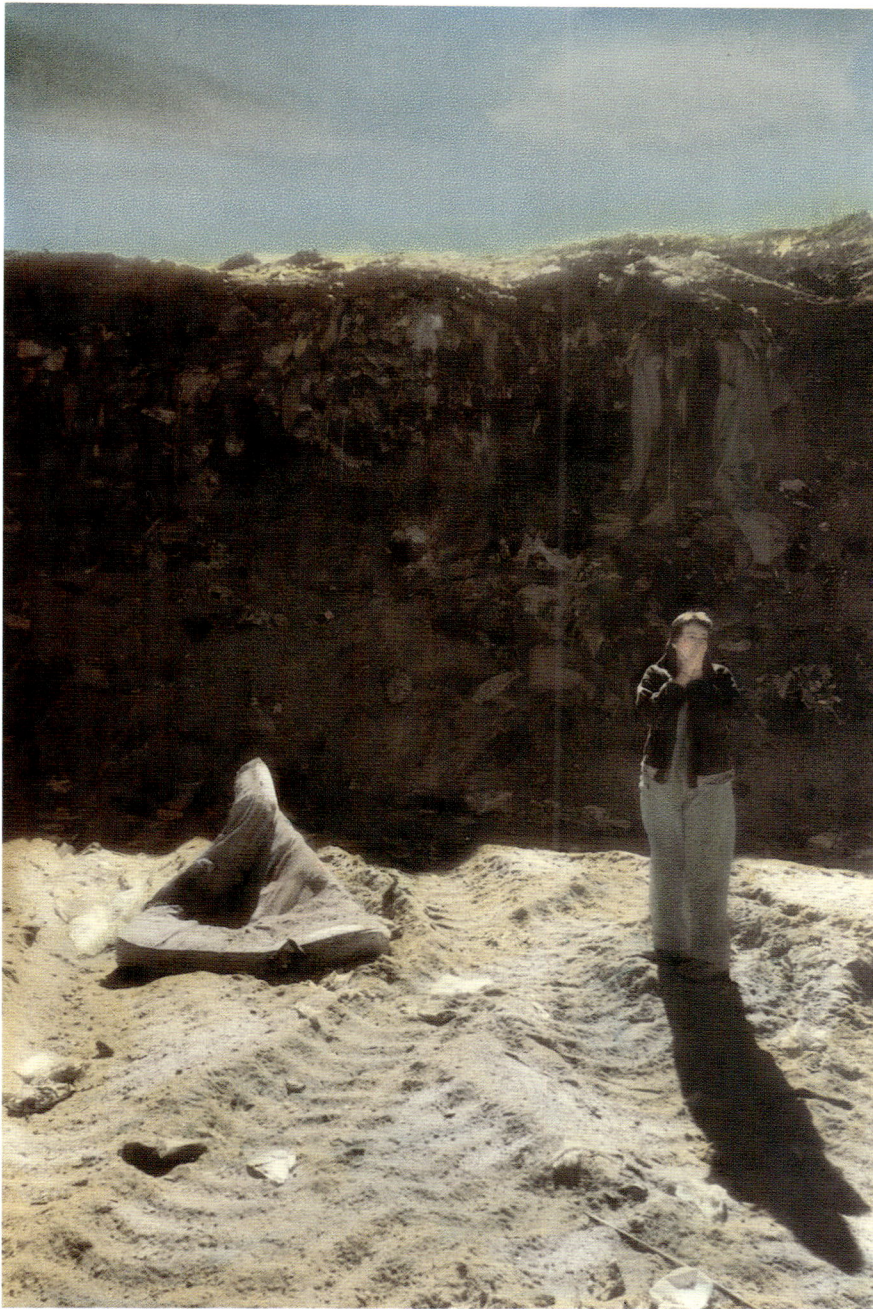

Kaolin

I WAS REPEATEDLY SEXUALLY
assaulted as a child by one of my
mother's boyfriends. After that,
I created a persona who was
worldly enough to believe
she had some control over the
sexual aggression of others.
But what had really happened
was that I had lost a part of myself,
the part that had known I was
worth more than an object.

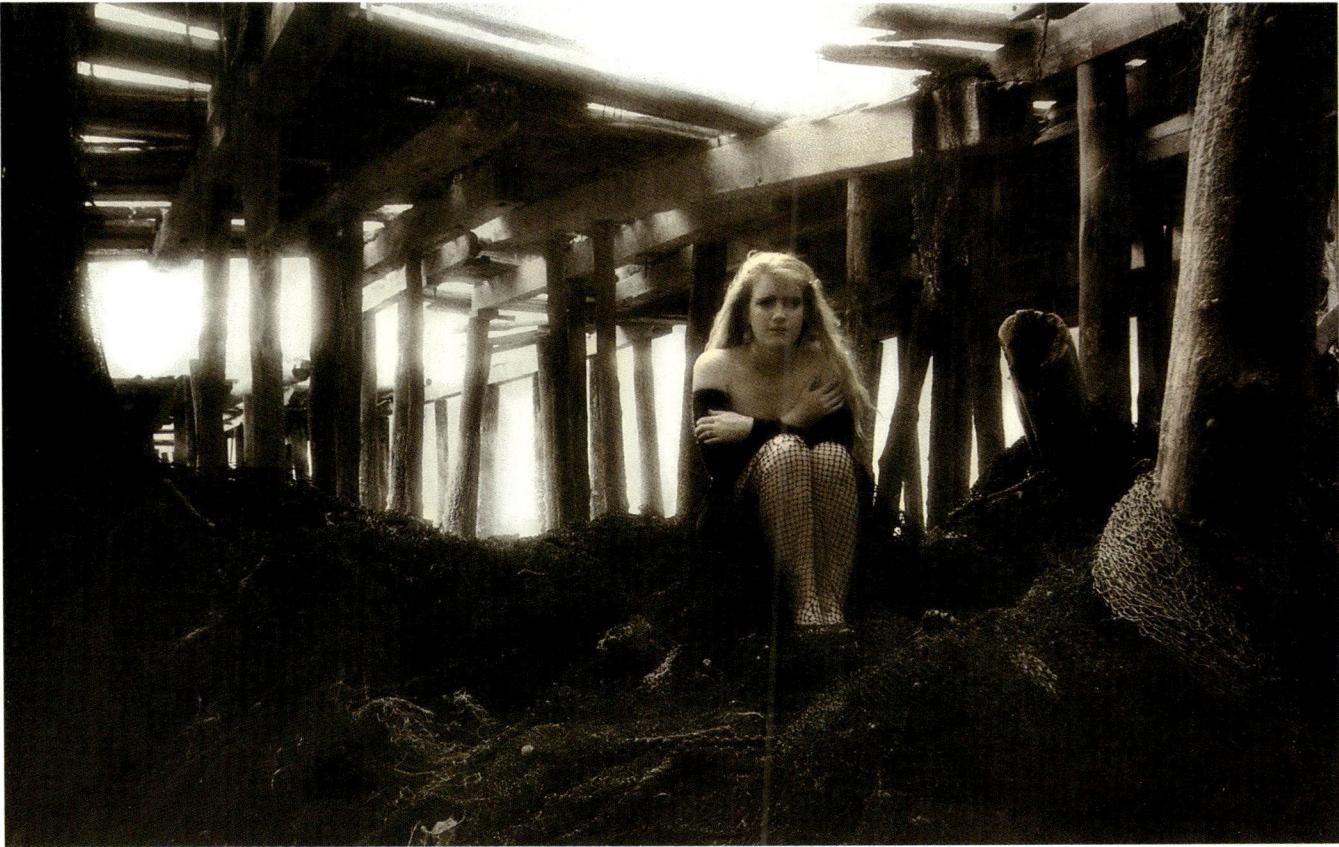

Khristine

THIS WAS THE ONLY DREAM

I remembered for many months.

I knew that I could walk straight

through that dark old house,

throwing open every door and

window, unlocking every cupboard.

My guide is waiting,

but am I willing?

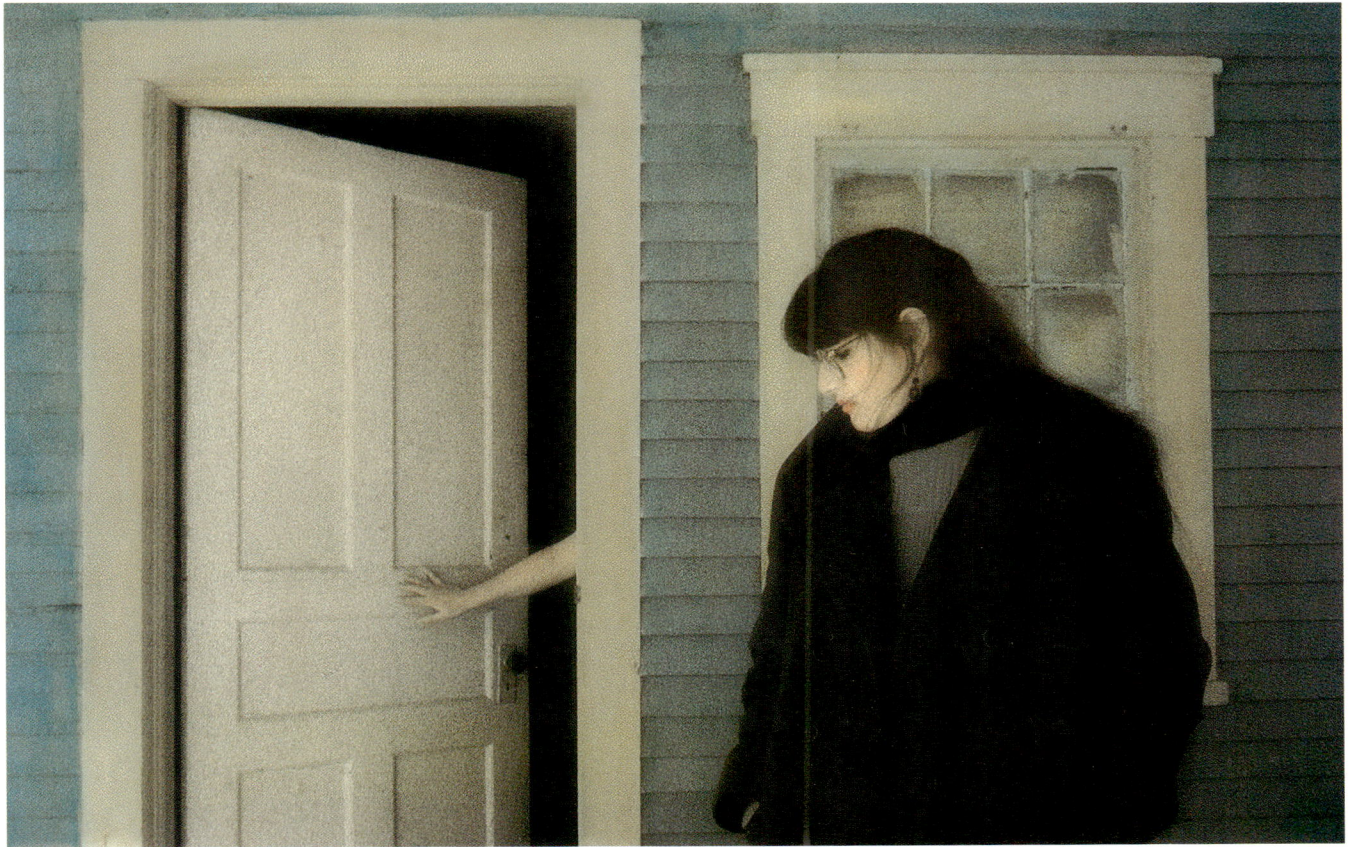

Yvonne

I AM SAD THAT IT HAS TAKEN

so much care to make this

one flower open. I want to feel

beautiful, and loved, and nurtured.

That shouldn't be so much to want.

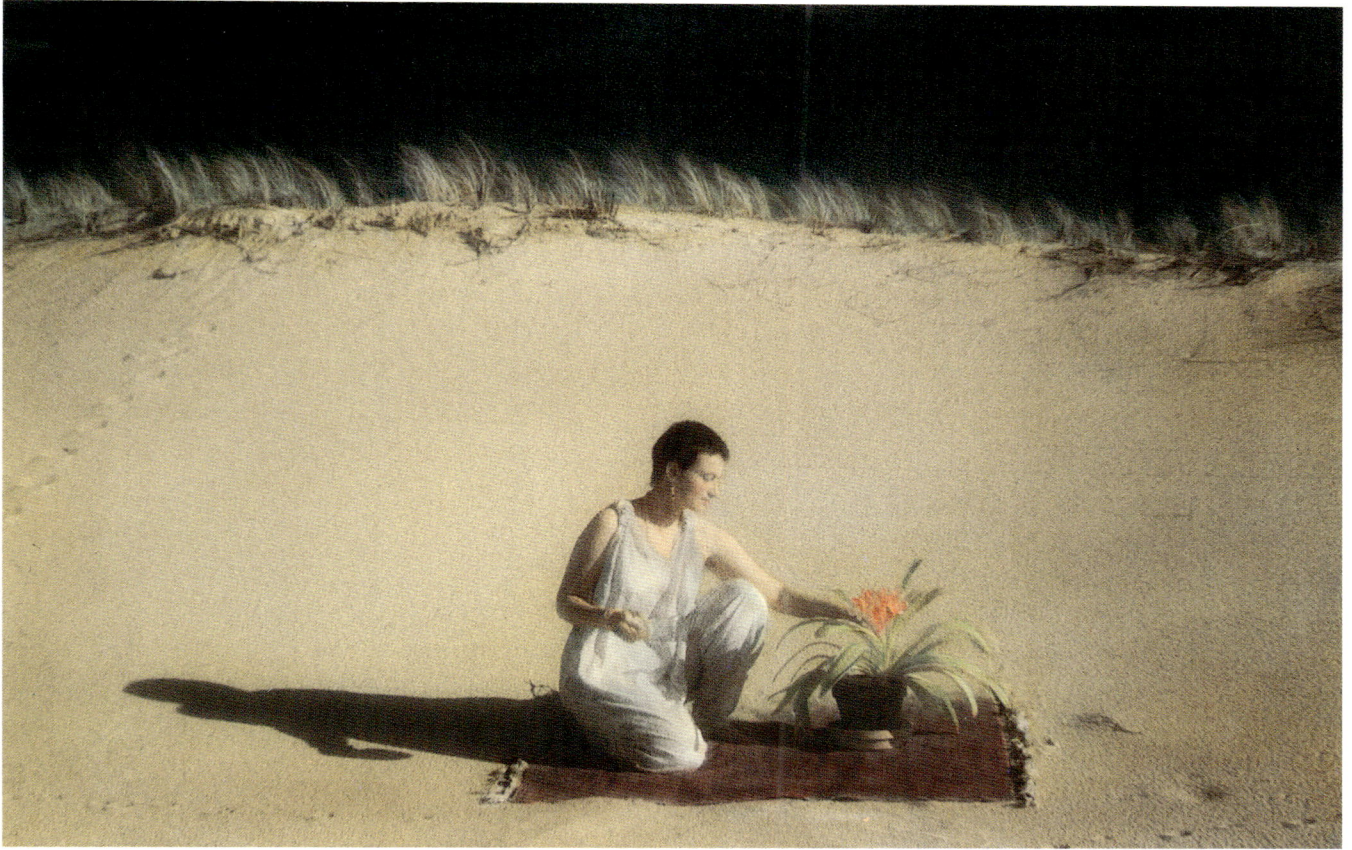

Patricia

The thing that hurt me

so badly became the catalyst

for my life's work. My paintings

are inspired by the deep pain

I have felt, and by my desire

to express it, transform it, and

finally let it go.

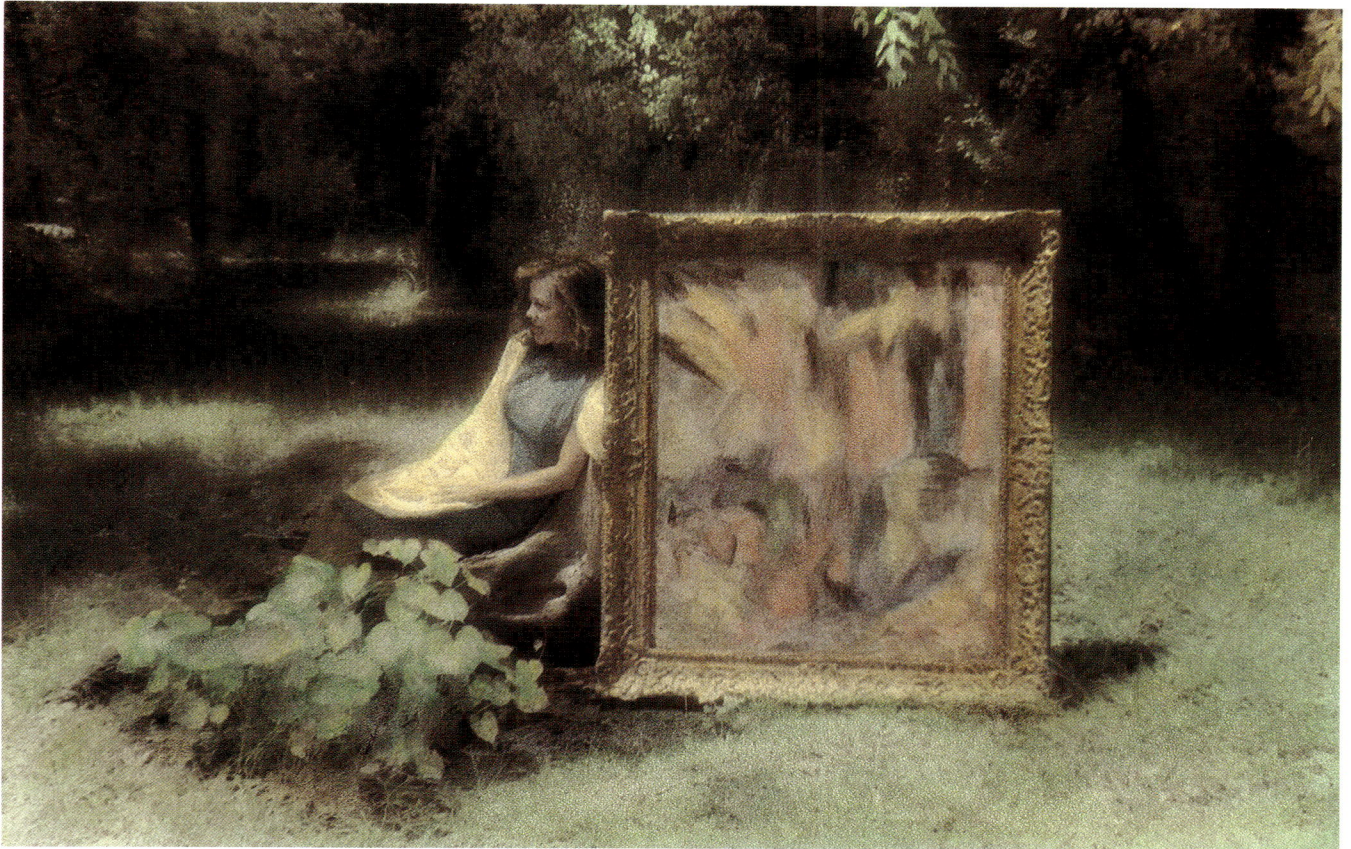

Khristine

If I close my eyes, I can

stand in the room where

my father died and run my hands

over the furniture. Sometimes

I can almost connect with him,

ask him why, even forgive him,

try to heal him too.

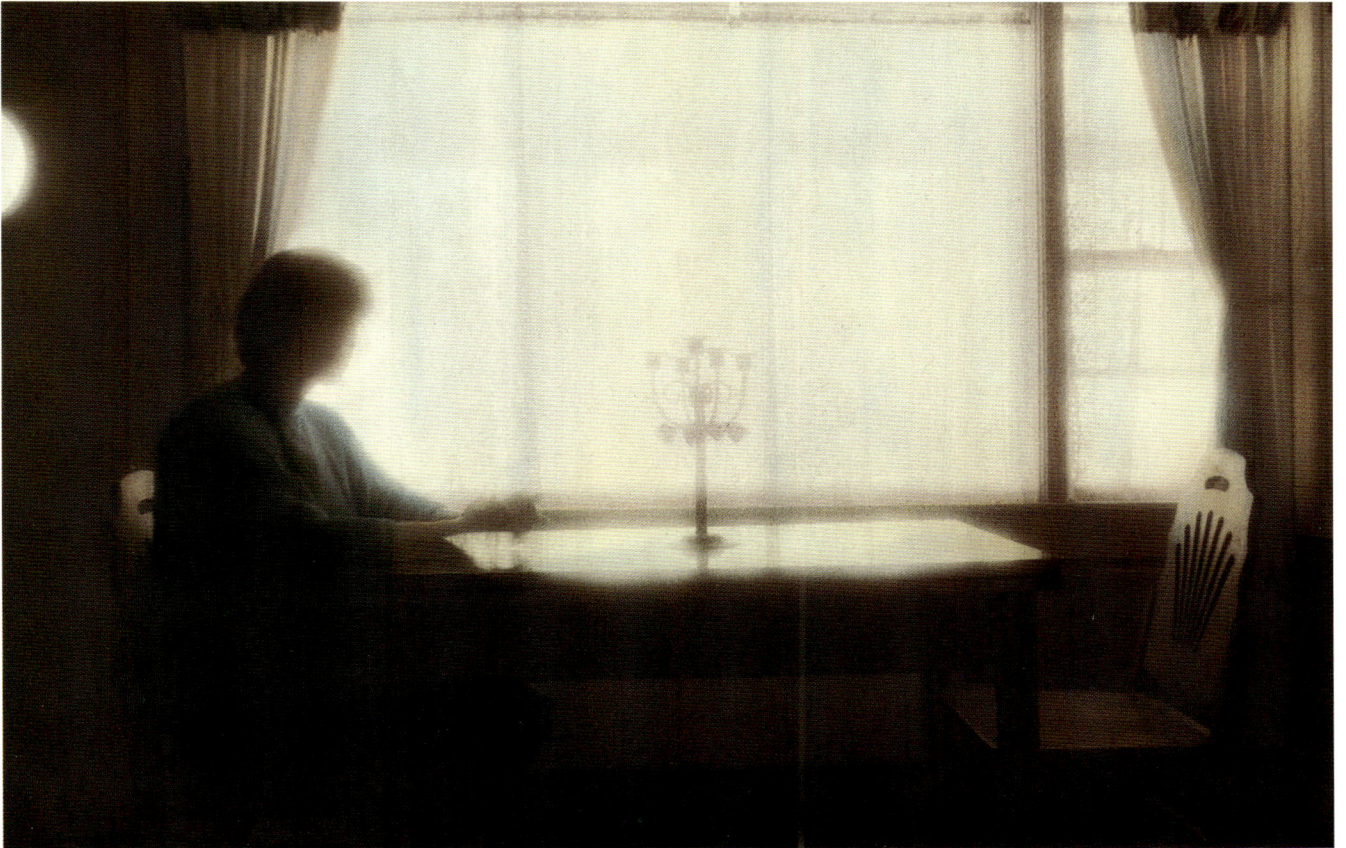

Liddy

We had a bittersweet meeting,

self and child-self. She has plans

to teach me about feeling free.

Then, if I could have one wish,

I would go back and relive

those lost years.

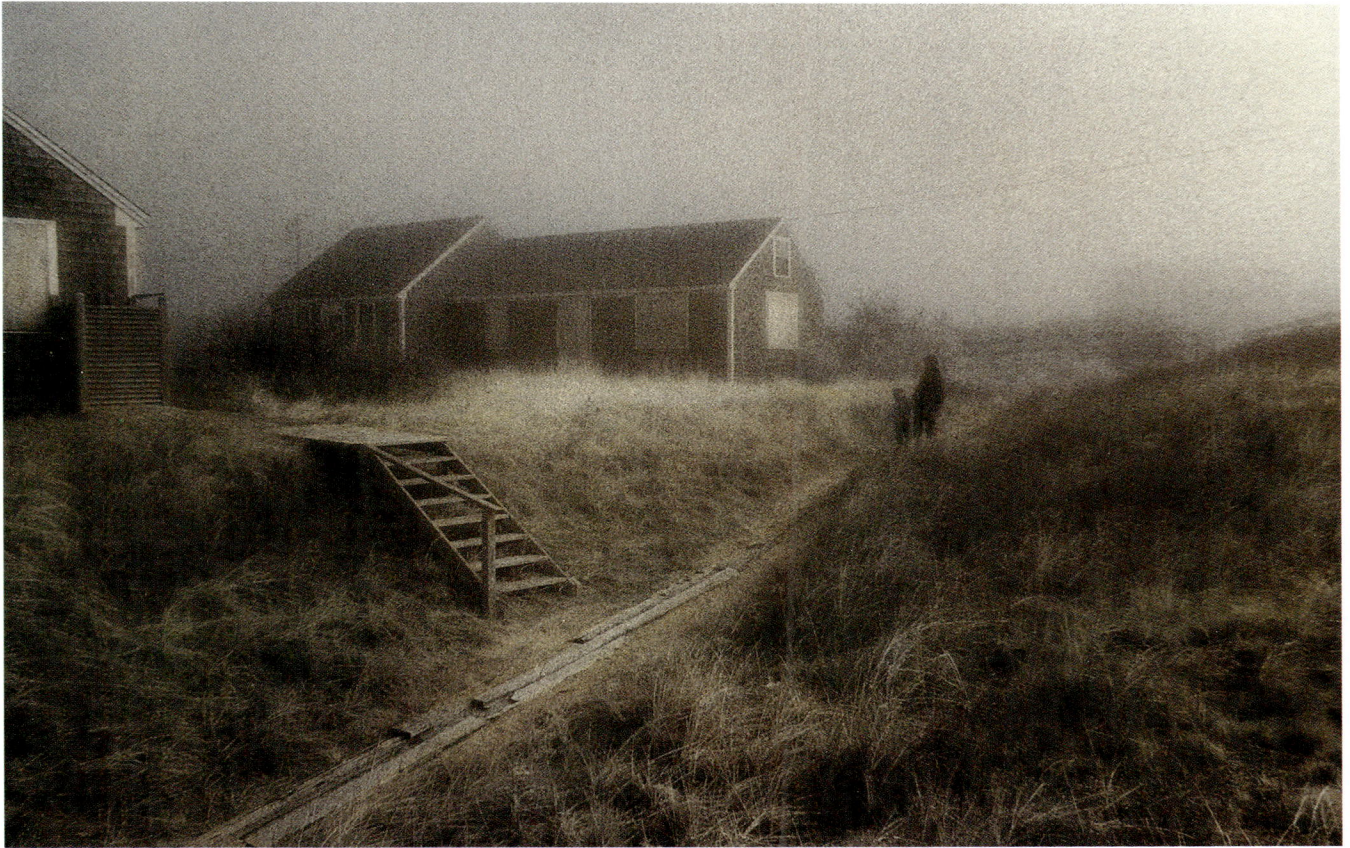

Mary

I was so tired of being in

hiding. Like a child, I needed

help to take my first steps out.

Now I feel warmth soaking into

my bones, nourishing my spirit,

and I'm glad. I've been in the dark

for long enough.

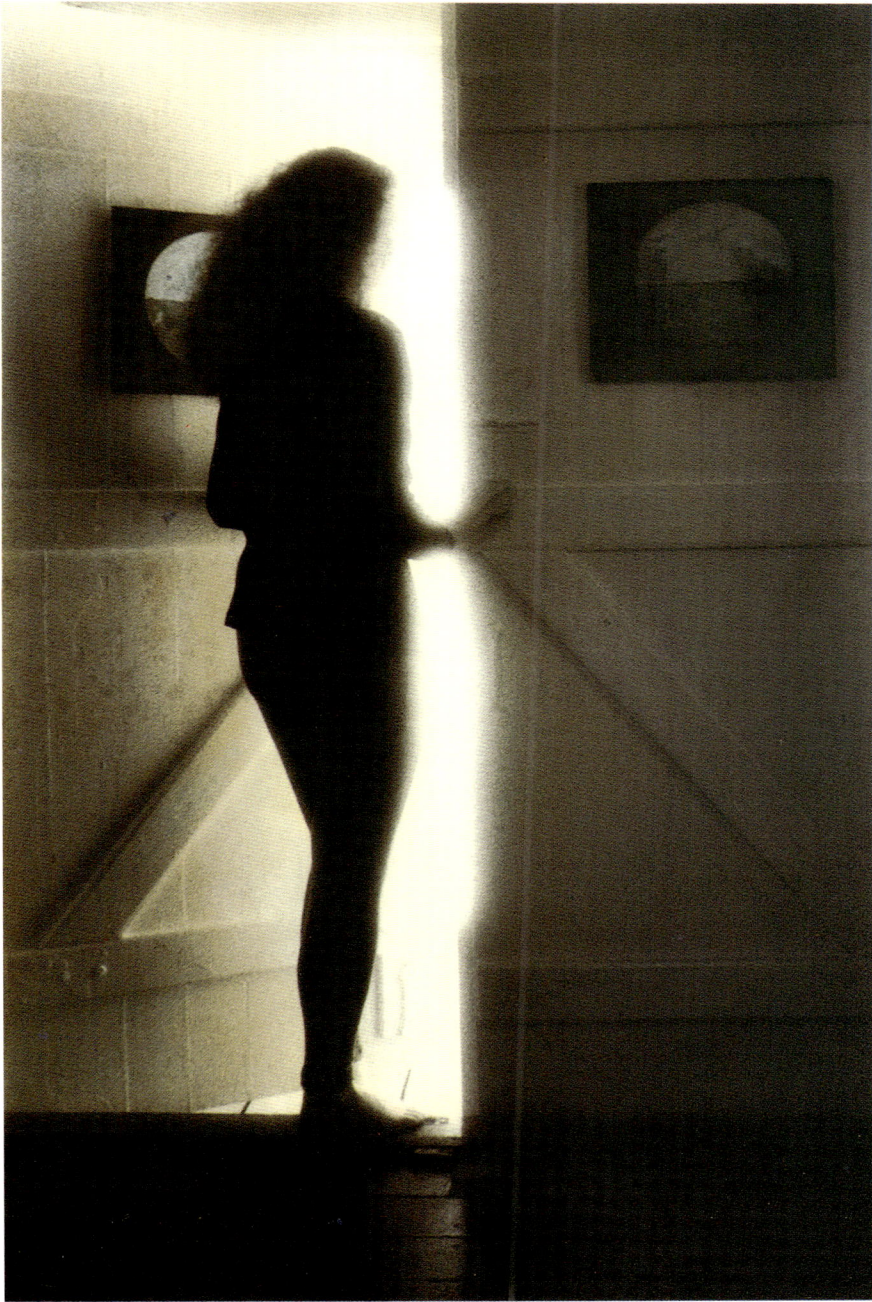

Kaolin

As a little girl, I loved to
spend all day exploring in the
woods and feeling at peace.
When suddenly the world turned
out to be crazy and dangerous,
I ran away to the only place I felt
to be safe and sane. Now in my
time of healing, I reclaim that
original bond with nature and
once again become a peaceful
child, filled with awe.

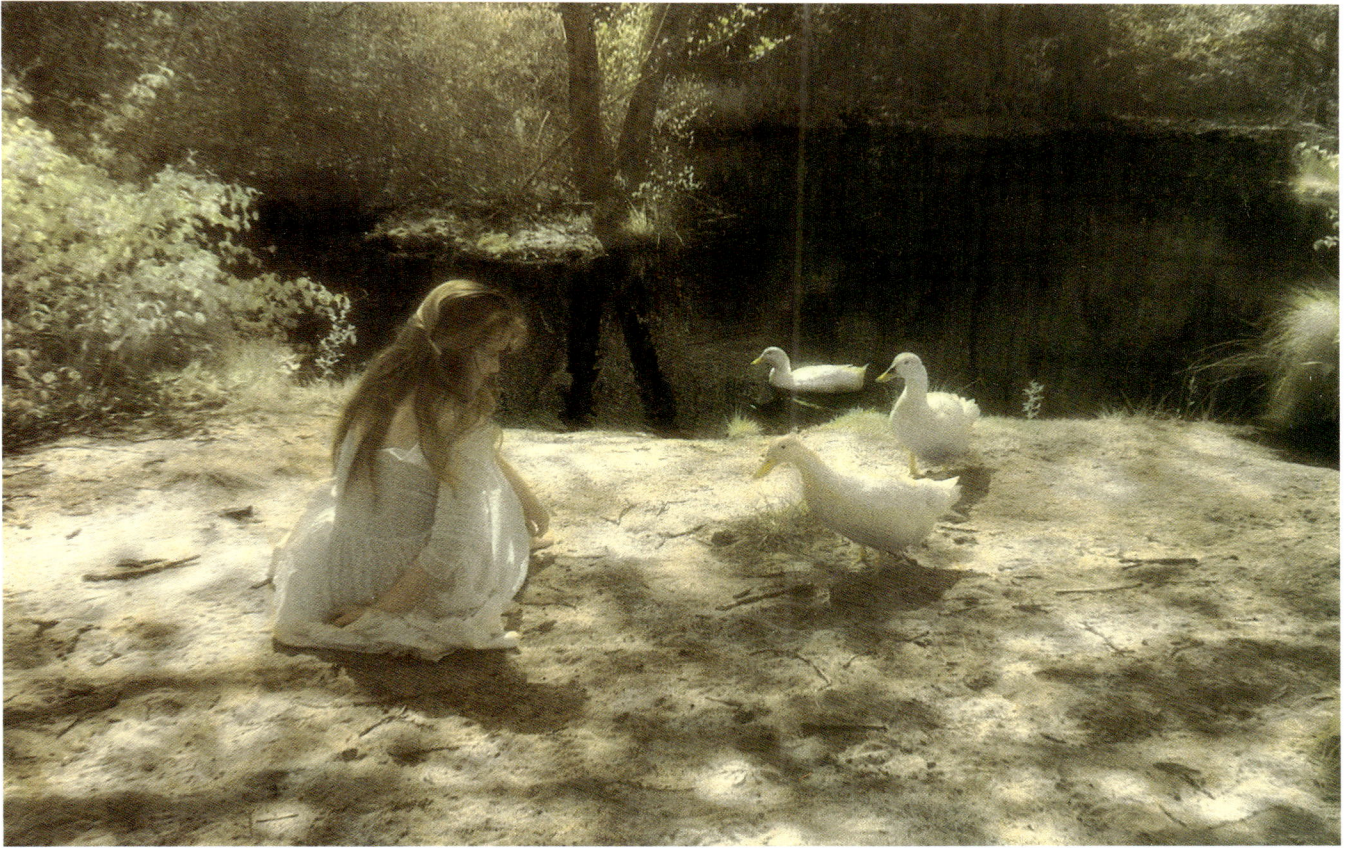

Nancy

SURVIVING ONLY MEANS ENDURING

in spite of the pain. In moments

like this one, the pain dissolves

as I accept and love the child I was.

Each encounter makes me stronger.

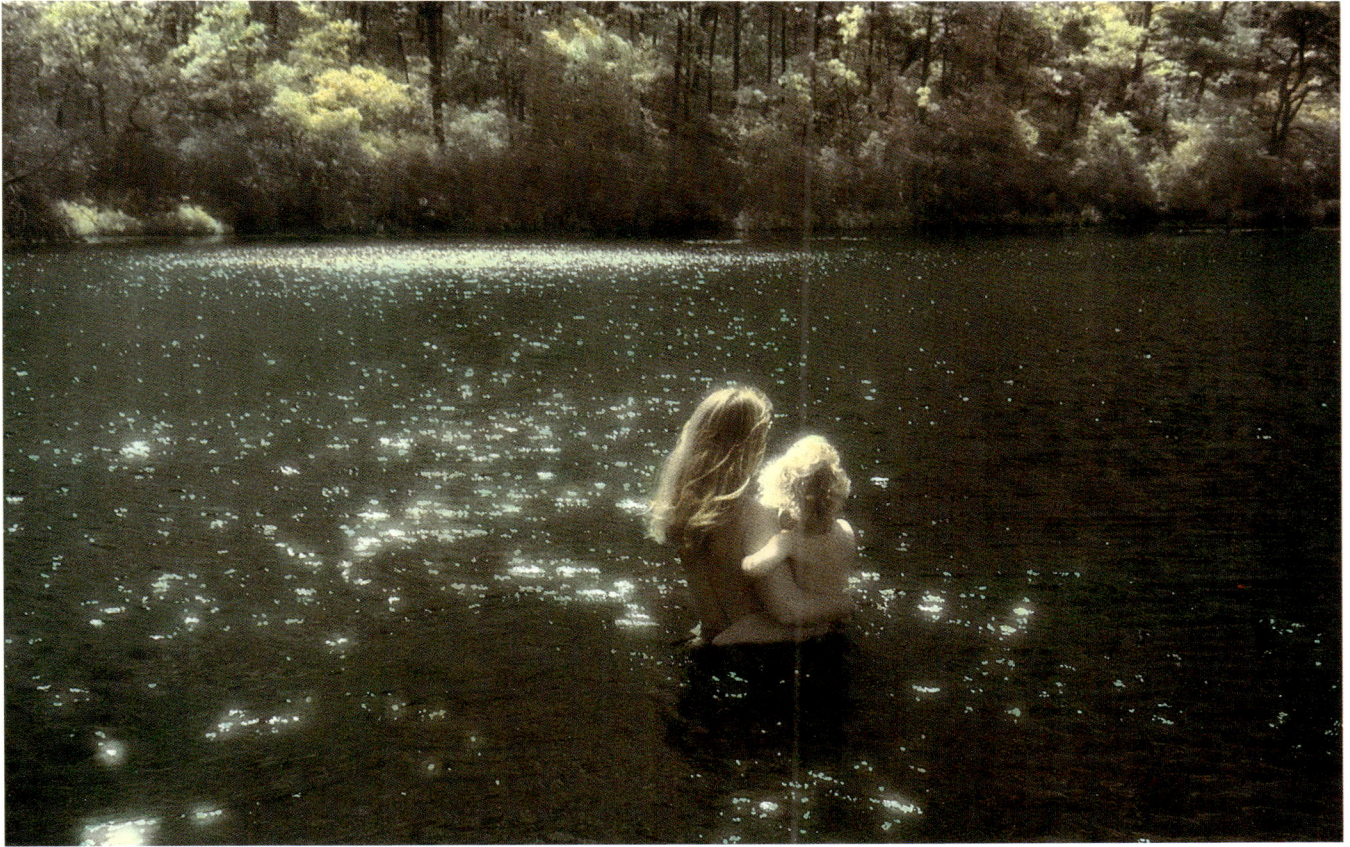

Epilogue

Healing at last,

we make a choice to

pass through the fire,

through the dark place,

to give birth to ourselves,

to parent ourselves,

to become whole.

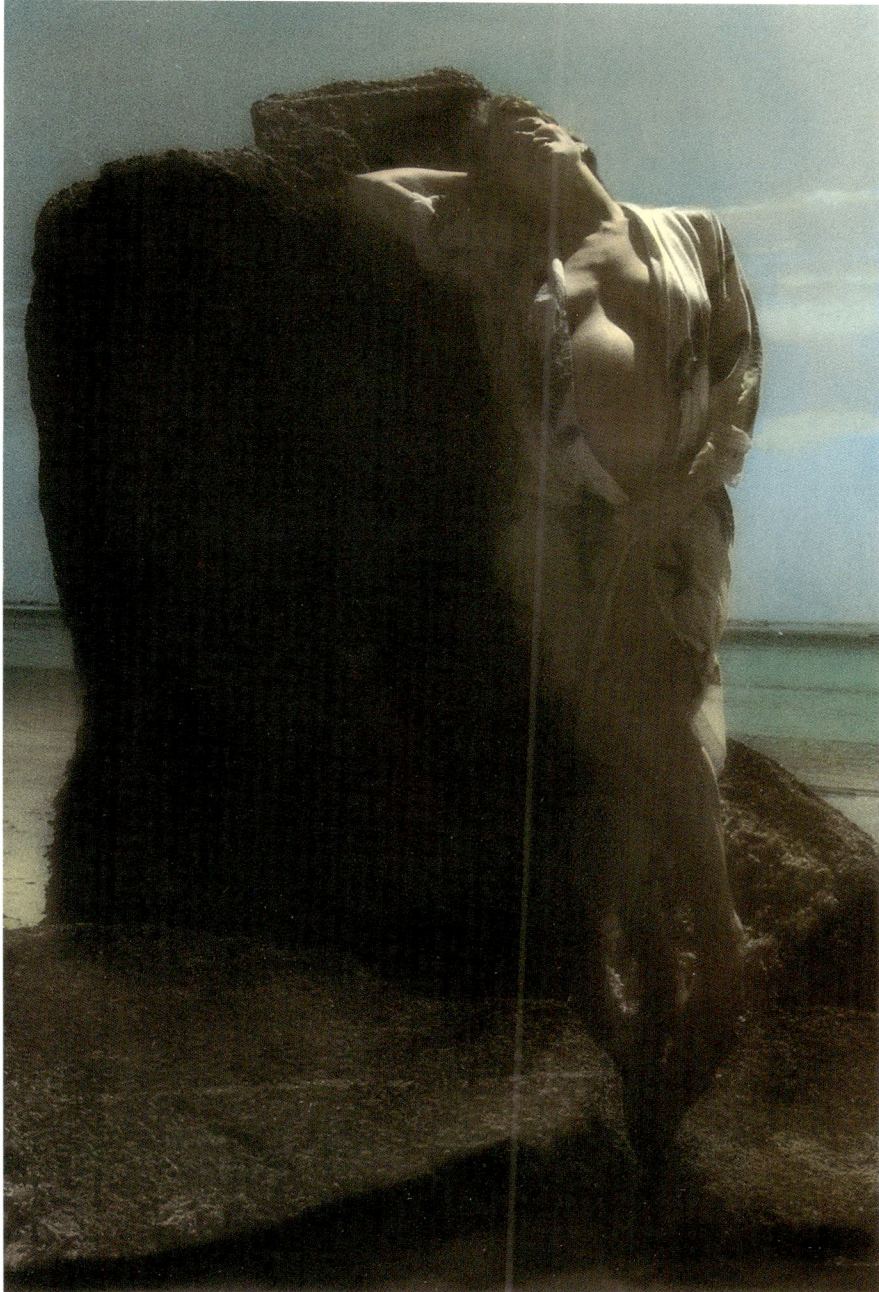

About the Author

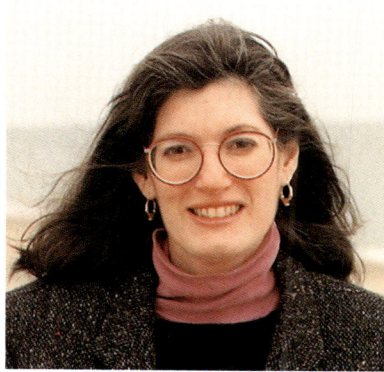

Photo by Danna Acker

Khristine Hopkins became enamoured of photography in 1976 while a student at the Exeter College of Art & Design, Exeter, England. After working for three years as a printer of black and white photographs in Western Massachusetts, she moved to Provincetown in 1980. The environment seemed to demand the use of color and she started to work exclusively with hand-coloring. Like many artists who settle in Provincetown, she draws much of her creative energy from her relationship with this beautiful place and the diversity of life which it supports.

Khristine lives on Cape Cod Bay with her husband, painter Donald Beal, and her son, Max Beal. She is Curator of Collections at the Provincetown Museum.

More books that can help

JOURNEY FROM BETRAYAL TO TRUST by Beth Hedva, Ph.D.

We are all familiar with feelings of betrayal in intimate relationships—whether from parents or significant others. This book distills the best of Dr. Hedva's workshops, blending ancient wisdom, stories, and myths with modern psychology to create concrete exercises and tools to help anyone who wants to exchange their feelings of anger and betrayal for a lifetime of trust and contentment. $12.95 paper, 224 pages

SELF ESTEEM by Virginia Satir

A simple and succinct declaration of self-worth for anyone who is looking for hope, positive feelings, and new possibilities about themselves and their lives. $6.95 paper, 64 pages

MAKING CONTACT by Virginia Satir

Drawing upon years of experience and observation, with a rich understanding of human potential, this beloved author shows us how to better understand and make contact with others. $7.95 paper, 96 pages

LOVE IS LETTING GO OF FEAR by Gerald Jampolsky, M.D.

The lessons in this extremely popular little book (over 1,000,000 in print), based on *A Course In Miracles*, will teach you to let go of fear and remember that our true essence is love. Includes daily excercises. $7.95 paper or $9.95 cloth, 144 pages

HEALING THE ADDICTIVE MIND by Lee Jampolsky, Ph.D.

The first book to use lessons from *A Course in Miracles* as a tool for overcoming addictive behaviors, including chemical dependency and codependent relationships. Includes daily excercises for overcoming harmful patterns and gaining spiritual peace. $9.95 paper, 172 pages

CLAIMING YOUR SELF-ESTEEM by Carolyn Ball, M.A.

A dynamic and practical guide to improving self-esteem. With powerful excercises, psychotherapist and teacher Carolyn Ball shows that when we learn to respect ourselves, we can live the kind of happy and creative lives we have always wanted. $9.95 paper, 224 pages

Available from your local bookstore, or order direct from the publisher. Please include $3.50 shipping and handling for the first book, and 50 cents for each additional book. California residents include local sales tax.

Celestial Arts
P.O. Box 7123
Berkeley, CA 94707

Also available: a videotape of **SURVIVORS**, narrated by Judith Israel with music by Dana Franchitto and Pat Metheny. The artist, Khristine Hopkins discusses the genesis of her project and the exhibition's emphasis on healing, 24 minutes. $21.95. Please include $3.00 for shipping and handling. Send check or money order to Tempest Press, P.O. Box 1438, Provincetown, MA 02657.